This book is dedicated to my parents.

The greatest legacy we can
leave our children is happy memories,
love's best preservative.

Og Mandino

Spirit Immortal

A Doctor Experiences Immortal Spirit at Birth and Death

Samuel G. Scime, M.D.

Part I

The Human Condition

Chapter 1: ....The Emperor's Question............9
Chapter 2:...............Personality and Human Behavior..........17
Chapter 3: ....Perennial Questions..........25

Part II

Extraordinary Experiences

Chapter 4: ....Discovery in Medicine..........31
Chapter 5:...................................Patient Encounters..........37
Chapter 6:..................................Brushes with Death..........47

Part III

The Material World

Chapter 7: ....Universe..........61
Chapter 8: ....Physical Phases and Transitions..........67
Chapter 9:..Light..........75

Part IV

Spiritual Paradigm

Chapter 10: ....Losing Personality..........83
Chapter 11: ....Birth Spirit - Existential Spirit..........89
Chapter 12: ....An Existential Paradigm..........95
Chapter 13: ....A Better Humanity........101

Appendix

Love, Truth & Beauty..107
Invocation of Birth Spirit..110

Part I

The Human Condition

The Emperor's Question

Personality and Human Behavior

Perennial Questions

Those who cannot remember the past
are condemned to repeat it.

George Santayana

Chapter 1

The Emperor's Question

The roar of the engines was nearly deafening. Attempting to hear the pilot's commands the crew members of the B-29 pressed their hands against their earphones. The plane shuddered as the bombing turn was made placing the target, Yawata, the Pittsburgh of Japan, within range.

My patient, Stanley Levine, is telling me about his experience as a radar navigator on his last WW II flight.

The target appears in the bombardier's scope, the doors open and he releases the bomb cables. But something is wrong. Two live bombs are hung up in the bomb bay. The bombardier climbs into the open bomb bay doors and onto a small cat walk. He struggles to loosen them by hand and finally succeeds. Immediately the plane is hit by flack from the heavily defended target. Engine number four is on fire and the fire is spreading towards the fuel tanks.

Lieutenant George Keller, the pilot, puts the plane into a steep dive, with a heading towards safety in Okinawa, recently won from the Japanese. With the plane in flames and unable to stay airborne everyone bails out into the Sea of Japan. Lieutenant Keller was last to jump. Altitude too low, his parachute had no time to deploy, taking his life. The surviving crew climbed into life rafts and drifted in the sea for one week, until they were picked up by a Japanese fishing boat a mile from shore. It was August 14, six days after the Nagasaki atomic blast.

When it was learned that the surviving crew members came from a B-29 the angry villagers beat them. At dawn Japanese military took them blindfolded to a nearby army camp where an executioner with long curved sword, chopping block and basket was waiting. A horrible POW fate of crew beheading was about to begin when suddenly a Japanese lieutenant, Nobuishi Fukui appeared with written orders to take command of the prisoners.

After securing the crew's release he took them to a railroad station where there were many Japanese civilians more interested in listening to a radio broadcast over loud speakers than in the POWs. Later they learned that they were listening to the Japanese Imperial Emperor, Hirohito declaring the imminent surrender of Japan and end to the war. Lieutenant Fukui had prior knowledge of the Emperor's announcement that day and thereby was able to save the crew at the last minute. In his speech the Emperor tried to prepare his countrymen to accept "the unthinkable, the unendurable, the insufferable humiliation" which was about to happen to them, the occupation of a defeated Japan by foreign forces for the first time in history. Among his statements was a question which keenly spotlights the fundamental cause of the war and also expresses the core enigma of the human condition. His question, "If all men are brothers, why does the storm rage in the night?"

The human storm is pervasive, not only in war, army against army, country against country, but people against people. In this, the 20th century alone, about 160 million people have been killed in wars, more than all the previous bloody history of mankind due to the deployment of the terrible technology of war weapons. Even today about 40,000 people a day are lost in the approximately 50 local wars that continue to burn over the globe, killed at the hands of the sick military and political minds of war. Hitler, Stalin, Pol Pot are recent but their ruthless savagery was pre-dated by the romanticized military leaders of the past, Alexander, Caesar, Genghis Khan, Atilla, Napoleon and many others. The human storm has a long history. Hopefully the current generation which has access to visual documentation of the horrors of war may be able to appreciate a future deterrent.

What is it that happens in the mind of a man of war to make him a killer, a military criminal? I was able to evaluate a soldier of this kind when I served as an army doctor at the 6th army prison, the stockade at the Presidio, San Francisco. In this capacity I admitted, examined, and treated all new prisoners. One of them was a man in his early 20's who spoke with a British accent. Physically he was healthy and strong. The military police had arrested him in northern California for driving a stolen rental car which he had taken from New York City. While in New York he went into an Army Recruiting Center and volunteered for enlistment. The sergeant agreed to his demand that he be assigned to the Green Beret infantry in Vietnam when he told the recruiter that he had prior military experience as a paratrooper infantryman in the British Army. For the recruiter this man appeared to be a star in his monthly quota enlistments, however as an army formality he had to request confirmation documents from British Army headquarters, and so he informed the soldier to wait a few days in New York City. If British documents confirmed his military history he was told he could bypass United States Army basic training and proceed directly to Travis Air Force base in California in preparation for transportation to Vietnam.

For the soldier a few days became several days and he became very impatient, demanding to start service. Information received from the British army revealed the man's history. He indeed was a member of British paratrooper forces who had parachuted into Nicosia, the capitol of Cyprus, during the civil war between Greek and Turkish Cypriot factions in the early 1960's. The British forces were to achieve order in the capitol and suppress the violence so that a peaceful solution could be attempted.

Britain was the logical country for their mission because Cyprus had been under British administration for decades following the earlier collapse of the Ottoman empire.

Rather than suppress violence this man was a generator of violence. He killed several Cypriot combatants and then started killing unarmed civilians wantonly. British officers disarmed him, arrested him and then sent him back to England where he was court-martialed and later dishonorably discharged from the military. Guessing that his past was about to catch up with him the soldier did not return to the recruiter in New York, but instead stole a rental car in New York and drove to the area near Travis Air Force Base where military police sighted the stolen car and arrested him. He had intended to sneak aboard a military air transport plane at Travis which was bound for Saigon and from there attempt to infiltrate into the front lines of the war.

When he entered the stockade at the Presidio his manner was cool, controlled and alert. Since he did not appear violent or aggressive and said that he had prior experience as a short order cook he was assigned to duty in the stockade kitchen. Several nights later he was caught trying to crowbar his way out through the bars of the small kitchen window. Restrained in heavy leg and arm chains, he was transferred into solitary confinement where he stayed for several days. It was after this confinement that the man revealed the nature of his mind.

In Nicosia years earlier he had tasted killing for the first time and enjoyed it. It made him feel an emotional rush of power and invincibility. The screams of his victims, he said, intensified the scene as he fired. *"So what if people die,"* he said, *"everyone has to die sometime, forever ending the miserable insignificance of human life."* Like many in the world he believed human life is essentially meaningless, an accident of the universe and certainly there is no survival of the finality of individual death. In his childhood he witnessed acts and words of violence frequently and later he hurt and killed animals. With no guidance the violent child became the violent sociopathic adult. The minds of violent and sociopathic people are the source and cause of human evil, so prevalent in the world. These minds directly address the emperor's question.

War is only due to the greed and
lust for power of relatively small groups,
the conspiracy of the few against the many.

Albert Szent Gyorygi
Nobel laureate in medicine 1937

Man must evolve for all human conflict
a method which rejects revenge,
aggression and retaliation.
The foundation of such a method is love.

Martin Luther King Jr.

Chapter 2

Personality and Human Behavior

What is it that determines human behavior? The personality that one develops over the years produces a wide variety of human behavior, resulting from the external experience and internal perceptions and thinking of a human mind. Behavior is an external act of the mind motivated by an internal conscious or unconscious summation of feeling, thinking, and reasoning. Learning, memory, emotion, thinking, reasoning, sense perception and motor activities are all functions of various parts of the brain. With hundreds of billions of neurons (nerve cells) and trillions of nerve synapses (connections to other nerve cells) and innumerable molecules of chemical neuro transmitters, the human brain is the most complex system known in the universe.

The physical, electrical and chemical structures of the brain of each infant are born of the intricacies of DNA genetic action and embryo development. All other body organs and systems are formed in similar fashion. The newborn brain has many more synapses than an adult human brain. The natural advantage is that the newborn can adapt to a wide variety of birth environments. Nerve connections that are not needed to survive and thrive early in life are deleted from the developing vast neural network. Experiences and positive intimate parental nurturing interact to help produce a sound neural brain complex capable of gradually developing a healthy personality. In the case of the violent British soldier this scenario did not occur.

Multiple theories of personality have been proposed over the years. Personality can be psychologically defined as the distinctive characteristics and characteristic relationships that determine a person's interaction and adaptation to other people and situations. Psychiatrists and psychologists have classified and reclassified various theories and schemes of personality.

Some of the major theories are those of Sigmund Freud based on psycho-sexual dynamics and the internal conflicts between the id, ego, superego and the unconscious. Karl Jung expanded the concepts of the unconscious into two areas, the area of personal repressed life events and the area of a collective unconscious of archetypes. Harmony of the conscious and unconscious in the process of individuation makes a whole, healthy person. Jean Piaget contributed to understanding the area of child psychology and intellectual development in childhood. Eric Erikson proposed a psychosocial theory of personality formation which is dependent on crises, circumstances, forcing personal choice, and change of personality direction. Carl Rogers proposed humanism and used patient encounter groups to assist communication and personal growth. B.F. Skinner proposed a psychology of behavioral science and studied the situation in which behavior occurs, the behavior and its consequences. He stated most behavior is selected by the consequences of that behavior. Intention, purpose and expectation are essential elements of behavior. Genetics, personal history and immediate environment are the impetus for behavior.

Behavioral geneticists study the influence of environment and genes on variations of behavior and have utilized twin investigations to demonstrate a genetic component in personality trait theory. Core personality traits were studied in both identical and fraternal twins and identical twins separated at birth and raised apart in a study conducted by the University of Minnesota. The character traits studied were introversion and shyness versus extroversion, stable and unstable emotion, agreeable versus difficult attitude, conscientious and undependable character, open and closed thinking. It was found that shared and unshared environment together with genetically influenced trait tendencies could be traced to the sameness and to the differences in twin personality that were observed. No single gene was responsible for a personality or character tendency but rather was dependent upon a blend of many different genes. The blend of genes is determined at the moment of conception.

Personality and behavior are multifactorial. There are many elements still undefined and unrecognized. The recent use of new psychotropic drugs on disturbed personalities demonstrates that personality can be altered through their use suggesting that personality also has neuro chemical roots.

The current President of the Czech Republic, Vaclov Havel, has described much of recent human behavior in a way characteristic of his pre-political artistic background. He states, "For the last many years, people have been guided by nothing higher than their own appetites." The appetite for political, sexual, economic and social power is what drives some people and some nations to exploit others for their own self-centered purposes. Rationalizing their thinking, they seek control and satisfaction without regard to the havoc and suffering inflicted by their actions. In the extreme war results, but selfish conflict reigns widely in human affairs.

The human storm also applies to the psychological internal conflicts of individuals who cannot resolve opposing internal stresses. The Christian apostle Paul stated it another way when he wrote in the Book of Romans, "For I do not do what I want, I do what I hate." The letter of James in the Christian Testament states that we are all tempted by our own desires. Judaism teaches that everyone has two impulses, one to good and one to evil. Avoiding evil and doing good is a common element of all religions. "Do not hurt others, do not injure by thought or deed, utter no word to pain thy fellow creatures."

from Hinduism. "Hurt none by word or deed, be consistent in well-doing." from Buddhism. "Whatever good you do for others, you send it before your own soul and shall find it with God who sees all you do" in Islam. These are choices of free will for each person.

Recent studies of brain electrical activity suggest that there is an internal conscious decider which makes the choices to act or not to act upon a thought. Neuroscientist, Benjamin Libet, of the University of California, San Francisco, performed experiments utilizing a rotating spot of 2.5 cycles per second on a TV screen. The tested person is asked to consciously decide to bend or not to bend his finger and note the position of the spot at the exact moment he makes the decision to move. An EEG head electrode showed a 0.35 second increase in electrical potential of the brain before the intention to act was made and 0.80 sec before the hand movement actually occurred. Neurologically it does not take that long for a brain message to reach the muscles responsible for the movement. Libet states that the brain neurons were firing before they were ever conscious of a desire to act. It appears that the brain had begun preparing for movement long before the mind had decided to act. Some subjects could change their mind after deciding to act. During the last 0.15 seconds before the action should have occurred the person decided to stay motionless. The mind decider, the source of the will demonstrated it's presence this way. However it is biologically and neurologically unknown.

Other scientific studies exploring the process of consciousness have implicated some brain functions but a complete solution to the problem of consciousness continues to be elusive. Positron emission tomography (PET) scanning of the brain utilizes the metabolic activity of radioactively tagged glucose molecules to create a computer picture of the brain in action. Consciousness appears to be more widely spread out over the entire cortex of the brain. In comparison, attention to visual or auditory signals is more localized to the areas of the cortex primarily responsible for those perceptions. It has been suggested that the synchronous and rhythmic firing of neuron layers of the cortex at 40 hertz oscillations per second are responsible for conscious attention to sensory signals. Alzheimer patients typically show reduced memory and confused attention to their environment. These patients have marked impairment of their PET scans and MRI scans (magnetic resonance imaging) particularly in the area of the prefrontal cortex. This area has been associated with working memory. The brains in these patients demonstrate atrophy of the cortical brain tissue. Scientists Dr. Francis Crick and Christoff Koch suggest that all aspects of the mind, including conscious awareness may be explained by the behavior of large sets of interacting neuron networks. This materialistic explanation emphasizes the intimate connection between neurophysiologic processes of the brain and the mind. But can it adequately account for the subjective experience of an inner self? Dr. Libet's experiments suggest otherwise. There is an internal decider suggesting a non material source of the experience of an inner self.

The only thing that makes sense
is that we are reborn.
We are reborn because it is
more interesting that way.

Norman Mailer

Chapter 3

Perennial Questions

The apparent meaninglessness of life and finality of death have been commonly held ideas in secular society. Such a belief produces anxiety and discomfort in people, at the least. Humanists create an arbitrary and relative meaning for life by centering on mankind's capabilities and values which results in human dignity. Nothing beyond the human level is required for understanding and acceptance. Many different schemes have been invented and designed by philosophers over the centuries in an attempt to neutralize the anxiety produced when the perennial questions are asked. "Who am I? Where did I come from? Why am I here? Where am I going? What is the meaning and purpose of my life? And of existence?" Many find comfort and strength to live their lives in accordance with religion. Some find help in understanding the psychological workings of the mind. Some scientists explain it as the critical anxiety of a vast neural network within the brain. To contemplate the existential questions privately is almost academic, but to experience them personally, in stark reality is quite another.

I was asked one day by the Chairman of our Ophthalmology Department, Dr. Charles Addington, to prepare interesting and challenging patient case presentations for a visiting Professor of Ophthalmology, Dr. Edward Maumanee. Dr. Maumanee held the chair for the Department of Ophthalmology at Johns Hopkins University Medical School. Thinking about patients who could be presented I decided to assemble a file on a new patient recently admitted, a boy of six with retinoblastoma. Retinoblastoma is the most lethal eye tumor of childhood. Many patients have a positive family history that can be traced. Some patients have no traceable family incidence and therefore are considered to have no genetic inheritance. They are considered to have sporadic and spontaneous cancers produced by unknown forces damaging the fetal retinal germ line. The cancer kills by spreading along the optic nerve and into the brain.

Mrs. Brown's child, the patient, had one eye removed three years previously for retinoblastoma. Now he was admitted to Roswell Park Memorial Cancer Hospital in Buffalo because of the discovery of retinoblastoma in his previously healthy remaining eye. Bilateral retinoblastoma is devastating for patient, parents, and doctor. At best, Mrs. Brown's child would be blind in his remaining eye if he could be treated by nuclear radiation. Effective laser treatment or photocoagulation was not yet developed. This eye also might have to be removed if it appeared that there was extension of the tumor into the optic nerve. Mrs. Brown's cries of anguish filled the hospital corridor.

She beseeched God loudly and angrily why her innocent child should have to suffer this way. For her, the existential questions were questions of terror. No doctor could soften her pain. Explaining that medical science had conquered many diseases, many natural evils, but not this one, was no help to her. I decided not to expose them to any more stress by including them in a clinical pathological conference. My ardent wish for them was that someday they would all find peace.

Carl Jung, the eminent psychologist, said that all of his patients over the age of 35 had at the core of their psychological distress basically religious questions. Answers to the perennial questions could make peace of mind possible for many people. My hope is that what follows serves that purpose.

Part II

Extraordinary Experiences

Discovery In Medicine

Patient Encounters

Brushes with Death

Man enjoys working for and expanding
his knowledge and understanding.
If we understood all natural phenomenon
this dear purpose would disappear.

Eugene Wigner
"Physics Professor, Princeton University"

Chapter 4

Discovery in Medicine

Medical science has made great strides through the discoveries made in the 20th century. From the improvements in hygiene and sanitation to antibiotics and advanced medical and surgical procedures all have accomplished vast enhancements in the quality and longevity of life.

Some of the medical discoveries have occurred serendipitously, by fortuitous chance or accident. Sir Alexander Flemming had been a medical officer in World War I, who after completing military service decided to research the properties of the bacteria staphylococcus aureus. This organism was responsible for much of the infection and mortality suffered by the soldiers in that war. One of the laboratory dishes in which he was growing staphylococcus had dislodged its cover for a few days by accident. He noticed an airborne mold had contaminated the culture, killing off the staphylococcus that was in that area. Flemming recognized the significance of his find and identified the mold as a strain of penicillium. Others then isolated the active substance which he named penicillin. In 1928, the antibiotic era began that day, in Dr. Flemmings's laboratory, caused by an accident.

Another example of serendipity or fortuitous chance is the discovery of anesthesia in 1842, by Dr. Crawford Long. While attending medical school at the University of Pennsylvania during the years 1838 - 1839, he was invited by friends to participate in a fraternity party. His friends asked him if he could bring along a supply of nitrous oxide, or laughing gas, for purposes of entertainment. They surmised that he might have access to it as he was a medical student. They were disappointed when he said he could not, but then he suggested a possible substitute. He told them that as a farm boy, growing up in northern Georgia, one of his duties was to clean the chicken coop with the solvent ether sulfate. When he did this he noticed that the chickens began to wobble about the cage uncontrollably, but recovered when the cleaning chore was over.

Since the chickens wobbling appeared similar to the staggering gait produced by nitrous oxide, he offered to bring some ether sulfate to the party if they wanted. That night a good time was had by all, with much laughing and staggering about the room. Some people fell, but then got up and continued with the festivities. The next morning, one of the men who had fallen was discovered to have sustained a broken arm without any knowledge of it or pain being experienced at the time of the accident. The man was treated with a cast and recovered, but Dr. Long remembered this event when he established his own medical practice in Jefferson County, Georgia a few years later.

One day in 1842, a man came to his office with a large abscess, or carbuncle, on the back of his neck. The medical technique of the day was to inebriate the patient by his consumption of alcohol, and then surgically open the abscess. However drunkenness, he told the patient, does not prevent the pain. He suggested ether sulfate as an inhalant substitute using the broken arm at the fraternity party as an example. The patient agreed to try it and Dr. Long drained the abscess without the patient feeling any pain. The era of general anesthesia was born that day. Dr. Long used ether again with several patients, including his own wife at her pregnancy delivery two years later.

Word of Dr. Long's discovery spread even though he did not publish it, and in 1844, dentist Dr. Horace Wells extracted a patient's tooth under ether. Then in 1846, Dr. William Morton removed an etherized patient's jaw tumor in the surgical amphitheater of Boston's Massachusetts General Hospital. He also reported ethers effects in the New England Journal of Medicine, which was the first public announcement of general anesthesia. Years later both men, Dr. Long and Dr. Morton, divided the $100,000 award Congress gave to the discoverers of general anesthesia. In addition, Dr. Long was given a Congressional pardon for being convicted and incarcerated for his participation as a Confederate Army surgeon during the Civil War.

The details of how major medical discoveries have been unexpectedly made in the past are surprising and interesting, but nonetheless true. I hope that the descriptions of my personal medical experiences which follows will permit similar interest, surprise, and consideration from you, the reader. However, my medical experiences are not in any way comparable to the momentous and unparalleled achievements described above. Dr. Flemming's, Dr. Morton's and Dr. Long's discoveries also have the great advantage of reproducibility within the scientific method which I readily admit mine do not. *Nonetheless, the following medical events are all true experiences.*

A soul? A soul is nothing.
Can you see it? Smell it? Touch it? ...No!

All That Money Can Buy
RKO Motion Pictures 1941

Chapter 5

Patient Encounters

My own personal experience has removed the question marks from the perennial existential questions and now I would like to share these experiences with you. These are three clinical encounters with three patients, one birth and two deaths, that taken together provide many answers.

The first patient encounter was with one patient who became two, an everyday miracle known as a birth. I was the obstetrical assistant for Dr. McDonald when he brought his patient, Mrs. Lo Bue, into the delivery room. It was during the summer of 1961, in Milwaukee Lutheran Hospital at Milwaukee, Wisconsin, that a newborn baby girl came into the world. I stood to the right of Dr. McDonald as the patient was placed on the delivery table. The mother's cervix was fully dilated and the baby's head was already at the beginning of the birth canal, but not yet presenting. I adjusted the surgical lights to focus upon the perineum and suddenly a violet circle of light appeared, centered on the bulging perineum as the baby's head started to descend.

Since I could no longer see the normal white surgical light I looked back to see if it was on or not and instead saw a broad beam of luminous particles flowing down straight over Dr. McDonald's right shoulder and into the baby's head at the birth canal opening. It continued to flow until the entire baby was delivered and I observed it during this time. It was not a uniform beam of particles as they were not all the same size and color. I gingerly leaned over so that my right eye entered the beam and I saw that the outermost particles were light pink in color, fuzzy, less discrete, and more macular in form and they flowed slowly. A feeling impressed upon me, the feeling of soft physical emollience, similar to what you feel when you slip into a warm bath on a cold night. These particles also induced in me the feeling of emotion, no one particular emotion, just generic emotion and desire.

As I moved my head further into the beam I encountered blue-colored particles. These were well formed and more compact than the pink and stronger with a feeling of power in each particle. They moved more quickly than the pink particles. The feeling induced in me was one of intelligence and knowledge. I moved my head and I entered the center of the radiating beam where I encountered very fast moving, very small discrete silvery white particles. They were very powerful and caused pain in my eye. I backed off quickly and could discern no feeling induced in me except that of awesome power.

When the baby was delivered the radiating flow stopped but there remained a large opening in the ceiling in the back of the delivery room which was the outside wall of the third floor delivery area and had no windows. I saw that a dark gray stirring wave was slowing down as it stirred a very large area of innumerable particles, suspended in a resilient pliable background. The wave moved counter-clockwise and I attempted to see the center of rotation by moving to the far left hand corner of the delivery room. I was unable to see the center point because the wave extended beyond the opening in the ceiling which moved in three dimensions while I moved to my left. Each particle embedded in the groundwork flashed a bright light as it rotated slowly on its own axis. It reminded me of the flashing light on top of a lighthouse. The hole in the ceiling gradually became smaller and smaller. Somehow I made time to assist Dr. McDonald with the episiotomy and the tying and cutting of the umbilical cord. Dr. McDonald, the anesthesiologist, and the nurses were all, I am sure, happy to leave the delivery room as I continued to watch the ceiling hole recede, and the normal ceiling reappear. I looked about the room to see if any reflecting object could have been the cause and found none. I inspected the surgical light and found nothing unusual about it. Then I left the room. No one questioned me about my actions as everyone left me alone.

As I turned the event over in my mind I was sure that my perceptions were not flawed and that the event really happened. I decided to go back to the delivery room to check again into the possibility of perhaps imbedded reflecting crystal-like material in the ceiling had caused it. I quietly slipped back into the now empty and unused delivery room and turned the lights on so that I could look closely at the ceiling. As I was looking at the back half of the ceiling a nurse came in and asked what I was doing and I explained that I was looking for anything unusual in the ceiling and asked her if she saw anything there. I pointed to the by now small point of light remnant of the ceiling hole and asked her what did she see? She said she saw a very small point of light but didn't know what it was. We both looked all over the ceiling for imbedded material capable of reflecting and neither of us saw anything else unusual. The next day the ceiling was intact with no point of light or unusual material in that area of the ceiling which had been effected the day before.

My next encounter occurred during the New Year's holiday season in 1962 at Milwaukee County Hospital. I was a member of a grand rounds medical team on the

Internal Medicine service at the hospital. We entered a patient's room in the older section of the hospital. These rooms had very high ceilings, roughly 10 feet high, no windows and a small single central ceiling light fixture. On the bed was a very frail elderly woman in a coma, Mrs. Walczak. An intravenous line was running and a Foley catheter was in place collecting her urine. She breathed very slowly, almost without movement and appeared to be in a deep coma. I stood at the far end of the room against the wall, facing the foot of the bed since others were conducting the examination of the patient. The Chief Internal Medicine resident physician then asked Tom, another member of the grand rounds team, to recover the urine collection bottle and take it to the laboratory for analysis. He disconnected the end of the Foley catheter from the large glass bottle sitting on the floor beneath the bed and proceeded out of the room with it. As he entered the threshold doorway of the room he tripped and the bottle shattered very loudly when it hit the floor. Mrs. Walczak suddenly startled, took a deep final breath and expired.

Within a few seconds a fine mist rose from her body. Misty particles from her legs, head and arms had flowed over the surface to meet around her upper abdomen and lower chest area and then rose towards the ceiling all together. The particles were swirling in great turmoil about 2 feet below the ceiling, directly over the body.

After several seconds the swirling stopped and the fine misty particles had coalesced into larger, less numerous, but very luminous particles. There then appeared to be a cloud formed above the patient and remained there for a few seconds. While the other members of the team were attending to the patient's body on the bed, trying to revive it, I was looking not at the patient but at the cloud that had formed above the patient. The cloud started to move towards me with pseudopod-like movements and quickly surrounded me with a feeling of presence. It was similar to being in a mid-winter blizzard with white-out vision; I could not see through it.

I reflexly felt threatened and mentally shouted "Stop!" Immediately the cloud presence receded to the foot of the bed. A few seconds after collecting there it proceeded to disappear luminous particle by uniform particle into a small area of space a few feet above the bed. Mrs. Walczak could not be revived and she was pronounced dead.

My last encounter occurred the winter of 1966, at Millard Filmore Hospital in Buffalo, New York where I was a resident physician. Late one night I was called to see a very ill patient on one of the Internal Medicine floors. Mrs. Romanello was an unfortunate woman in a coma, dying of metastatic breast cancer. She had difficulty breathing and the Levophed intravenous line was not able to sustain her blood pressure in an acceptable range. I sat on the left side of the bed while I leaned over her and applied a stethoscope to her heart. Her heart rate was slow and of feeble intensity. Her anterior lung fields were full of the crackling sounds typical of atelectasis (lung collapse) or worse, lungs filling with fluid. While I continued to examine her she expired. I could hear no heart beat, just silence.

Within a few seconds, a fine mist rose from her body hitting me on the left side of my body as I was leaning over her. I immediately pulled myself off the bed while turning my body to the left, trying to avoid more mist coming off her body. The mist particles accumulated into a cloud at the foot of her bed where it formed into homogeneous large luminous white particles. These then disappeared into the air particle by particle. For years I felt a fine tingling sensation over the left side of my body through which the initial mist passed. I had no loss of coordination or muscle strength or movement and the sense of touch in my left hand remained normal.

Analysis: These three cases are related. In the case of the first and the third patient I saw and physically felt the spiritual particles entering the body at birth and leaving the body at death. In the second patient, Mrs. Walczak, the spiritual cloud formed at death demonstrated intelligence and purpose of movement reflecting qualities of mind and will. The birth spirit enters from another unseen dimension of existence and leaves at death to pass into a comparable unseen dimension. The spiritual energy at birth is originally not homogeneous, consisting of a combination of soft pink fuzzy energy, blue stronger more defined energy particles, and very strong powerful small white spiritual particles. But the spiritual energy that leaves the body is homogeneous and luminously white. Within the journey of a human life a spiritual transition takes place. With all of life's ups and downs, stresses, successes and challenges, human life has a purpose; the changing and evolution of a spiritual being who exists and survives death.

Miracles happen,
not in opposition to nature,
but in opposition to
what we know of nature.

Saint Augustine

Chapter 6

Brushes With Death

I have experienced closeness to my own death many times. The Angel of Death first appears to be terrible. Fear is a natural response, but as death approaches closer I felt it to be a trusted friend and learned how to surrender to it. One of my earliest experiences with it occurred during the winter of 1957, which was particularly good for snow fall. At that time I was an instructor in Comparative Anatomy at Canisius College in Buffalo, New York. The chairman of the Biology Department, Father John Frish, S.J., appointed a new instructor each year from the biology majors. The appointee was compensated with a half-tuition scholarship. The senior instructor for that year was John, from the class before me.

One Winter day he invited me to accompany him and a group of his fellow classmates on a skiing trip to Honey Harbor, Canada, where one of the seniors' family had a summer fishing cabin on the shore there. Honey Harbor is about 150 miles north of Toronto at the edge of Georgian Bay. If you look at a map you will see that Georgian Bay is an eastern extension of Lake Huron. The drive from Buffalo to Toronto was about 100 miles and I was concerned about my car making the winter trip safely. After settling into the cabin at Honey Harbor upon arrival we prepared for the skiing and tobogganing trip the next day. We walked to the area with skis on our shoulders and dragging toboggans. It was a cold, but bright sunny day and the area we walked to was very good for skiing and tobogganing, having no trees and gently rolling hills. We all had a great time skiing and tobogganing there, so much so that we lost track of time.

The sun was low on the horizon before we realized we should start back to the harbor. The walk back started out fine. I was pulling a toboggan, but after a while the afternoon's exertion caught up with me and I ran out of pulling energy. Someone else took the toboggan and I continued on. We were all in a sorry state of tiredness and started to separate out, each according to his own physical reserve. A while longer, I found that I could not keep up trudging through the snow and I lost sight of the rest of the group ahead of me. By this time I was onto a frozen lake. I was happy because I thought walking across the frozen lake would be easier than trudging through the thick snow fields. It was easier, but not that much easier. I soon became physically exhausted and felt that I had to rest awhile. I rolled over on the ice so that my face would be facing into the remaining sunlight in an attempt to keep myself from falling asleep, and also to orientate myself in direction, but it didn't work. After a fight to stay awake, I finally surrendered to a cold sleep. It felt like I was falling into the dark face of death.

After an unknown period of time my eyes opened spontaneously and I was shocked to find that night had fallen and I could not see my landmarks. I had regained enough energy to get to my feet and struggle on. I didn't know what direction I was headed for and felt that I was lost. I could be walking back towards the direction of the skiing field. As I groped across the frozen lake I searched for signs of life somewhere ahead. I still could find nothing. Then suddenly I saw a small glimmer of light far in the distance. Now at least I had a direction to walk to. As I stumbled forward towards the light it became more visible. By this time I was cold and shivering, unmistakable signs of the beginning of hypothermia, but I could still walk. It took several more minutes on the frozen lake until I reached the shore. There was the source of light, a small cabin in the woods with its outside bulb above the doorway radiating its life saving beam.

I rested on a nearby rock trying to regain strength and psychological composure before I went to the door. However, when I got to the door, I unconsciously began to pound on it. When the door opened, I fell into the doorway. There were a man and woman, occupants of the cabin, who helped me into a chair and gave me some hot tea. The hot tea and warmth of the cabin brought me around and I became aware that there were some other members of the skiing group in the room, each with a drained, exhausted look on their face. No one said a word. Later a truck came and took us back to Honey Harbor. The next day I drove the members of my group back to Buffalo.

No one said a word during the entire return trip because we all had faced death on that trip.

Another close call with death happened the summer of 1957. Between school semesters I wanted to earn money in preparation of school tuition. I was able to get a job with the Laborers Union as a construction worker with the Cowper Construction Company in Buffalo. They were building a multi-building apartment complex on Grider Street near the county hospital in Buffalo and my job was to help construct the concrete floors and ceilings of each level of one of the buildings. This was done by large cranes which lifted large buckets of wet concrete. Each floor was poured into a web of steel reinforcement bars held within the wooden and steel flooring forms. There are wood T joyce supports, beneath each new floor, supporting the large plywood sheets which form the bottom of the floor mold. When the concrete of the poured floor was set my job was to go beneath the new floor, remove the supporting T joyces and then the large plywood sheets. These joyces and sheets are then put together in groups at the side of the building, to be used again on the next floor pouring above. This required two men at either end of the long six foot plywood sheets, moving to the side of the building and flipping the plywood up over the side of the building, and onto the new floor constructed above. My team was on the fourth floor and the fifth floor pour above us was dry.

My partner was Ed Polakowski. He was ideally built for construction work, big and heavy. At the other end of the plywood sheet was me, a light 123 pounds. The first few sheets went well, up and over the side of the building and on to the fifth floor above. On the flip of the next sheet a sudden gust of wind came up, making the plywood sheet act like a sail. The force of the wind made the plywood twist in my hand and as I tried to re-grab it the force of the wind pushed me out over the open side of the building. Ed was anchored well on the other side of the sheet and shouted for me to try to work my hands back over the plywood and pull myself back into the building. I tried but couldn't do it, the wind was too strong. Looking down I saw the heap of broken concrete and rubble on the ground four floors below me and I dangled there helplessly. When Ed saw I couldn't move, with my left foot only on the edge of the building, he worked his way, hand over hand, across the top of the plywood and reached out and grabbed me by the belt and pulled me inside. Badly shaken, I just sat there and we both agreed that this was no job for me. Ed Polakowski saved my life that day.

My next close call came when I was a medical officer in the Army in Korea in 1963. My official title was Battalion Surgeon and then later Commanding Officer of the 150th Medical Detachment of the 8th Army in Korea. The Detachment consisted of two medical facilities, one on the army post in the Taejon Valley, another in the mountains high above. Taejon was the fifth largest city in South Korea and the

Taejon line was the first organized line of allied defense against the North Korean communist invasion of South Korea in 1950. My original assignment was as Battalion Surgeon to the forces in the mountain location, a high security post. Rarely was I able to leave the compound area, but on one weekend I was able to go to Seoul and stop at the Bachelor Officer quarters there.

That Friday evening I ate at the officers club a dish of Bulgogi and kimchee with rice. Kimchee is a Korean mixture of marinated fermented vegetables and Bulgogi, a thinly sliced, marinated Mongolian beef. I wanted to practice my chopsticks skills and while I struggled with it a Korean national approached my table and asked if he could join me and talk. He introduced himself as Mr. Park, and was a well-dressed man with a good command of the English language. He asked why I was eating a Korean dish and also with chopsticks since most Americans there were eating with the normal western utensils. I told him I was interested in learning about Korean food and culture. This impressed him and he began to describe his family, showing me a picture of his wife and children. Learning that I was a doctor based in the interior of the country and visiting Seoul for the first time, he invited me to come to his home and meet his family after dinner the following night. When I accepted his invitation he suggested a fine Korean restaurant called "The Korea House" which was located on the top of the Chosen hotel in downtown Seoul.

He picked me up the following night at the Bachelors Officers Club. He was driving a black car of a make I never saw before or since. After a hearty greeting I climbed into the front seat and he drove off into the early evening darkness. Down wide boulevards and side streets we went, past some small parks and temples and then into the area of downtown Seoul. Finally Mr. Park reached our restaurant at the Chosen hotel. He drove down a long narrow alley which opened onto a large spacious courtyard in the front of the hotel. The courtyard looked deserted and the hotel was at the far end. After a short way driving into the courtyard there suddenly appeared a large group of people with lighted torches in their hands. They quickly surrounded the car and started to rock it back and forth. The car engine died. The mob of people pounded all over the car. There was a terrible cracking sound as the windshield broke and I could see the yellow glowing lights moving all about the car. The car rocked from side to side as the mob tried to turn it over and probably set it on fire.

When I realized that I was facing a terrible death I heard and felt an internal clicking, a snapping sound, and immediately my mind and spirit rose up high, out of the car and above the courtyard. I could see the car in the courtyard and the surrounding yelling crowd with torches in their hands. I spun far above the courtyard into the dark sky and I was able to see the entire area of Seoul at night with all the glowing lights and buildings. A feeling came over me that everything would be all right and then I became aware of myself again in the car.

I looked over and saw Mr. Park turning the ignition key, desperately trying to restart the car. Another turn of the key and the engine started.

He then put the car in gear and accelerated forward racing across the courtyard, towards the far end, with the mob in pursuit. He slammed on the brakes and turned the car around in a skidding maneuver so that the car faced the only entrance and exit way to the courtyard. But the car stalled again after the sudden pivoting turn was completed. The mob rushed closer with torches ablaze. More frantic attempts to restart the engine and finally it caught. Mr. Park quickly put the car in gear again and raced forward, straight into the mob. In the few seconds it took to reach the mob the car was accelerating and I could hear bodies being hit as he drove through the mob to the entrance alley way. Mr. Park took me back to the Bachelors Officers Quarters and he returned home. Both of us were so shaken we didn't speak much except to say good-bye to each other.

The last brush with death occurred while driving to Florida in the month of February. The winter was particularly hard that year in Buffalo and I was anxious to start a weeks vacation there. I drove from Buffalo to Erie, Pennsylvania on interstate 90 and at Erie turned south towards Pittsburgh. This was a divided highway passing through the beautiful Allegheny Mountains. The weather started out clear that early evening in

Erie. But less than an hour later a blizzard started and grew in intensity. On the right side of the road were heaped up snow banks from previous snow plowing by the state, and on the left side of the road was an unprotected drop off into the valley below. There was a tractor trailer in front of me and I stayed behind it, using its red tail lights as a guide to the road. But crosswinds coming off the body of the trailer intensified the white out blizzard effect on my vision so I had to fall back.

After a while I found that the wheels on the right side of my car were caught on the gravel apron of the road. Visibility was poor as the blizzard continued to intensify and I thought I might hit a snow drift on the side of the road without seeing it. I tried to bring the right tires back onto the roadway and found the pavement lip on the right side too high to allow it. With what I thought was a mild jerk of the wheel to the left I lost control of the car which spun for several 360 degree turns. The lights of the cars behind me were coming through the windshield on each rotation. I felt that I was sliding off the far side of the road and down the unprotected drop off and was convinced that death was eminent. Suddenly I heard a soft internal click and immediately saw all the scenes of my life pass before me, starting with the most recent. The images were all physically vivid and emotional. I felt the pain and anguish I had caused others as if I were now the recipient. Embarrassing, difficult and painful experiences I had lived contained no emotion at all, just a neutral experience. Common, everyday and good experiences, which were all other experiences not included in one or two above, contained an intense emotion of joy and agape. Every event of my life was recorded in vivid reality. Then from some unknown source I heard a voice say, "You can get this car under control." I grabbed the steering wheel again which continued to freely ski without any road feel to it. I twisted the wheel back and forth. Miraculously the car began to straighten out and was back on the road and heading in the right direction. I had hit nothing in the process.

These experiences early on in my life intensely demonstrate to me not only my own physical mortality, but also the existence of a non-mortal self who helped me survive these brushes with death.

Part III

The Material World

Universe

Physical Phases and Transitions

Light

The most beautiful experience
we can have is of the mysterious.
It is the fundamental emotion
which stands at the cradle
of true science.

Albert Einstein

Chapter 7

Universe

Ancient people observed the night sky and phases of the moon and sun transits which helped them recognize good crop planting times, rainy seasons, flood threats and aided them in open water navigation. Creation stories were devised in many ancient cultures which allied insignificant and vulnerable man with the powerful and beneficent forces of nature. Early nature religions of Babylon, Egypt, Greece, India, China, and other cultures claimed divine origins for their ancient concept of universe, creation from gods, Babylonian and Egyptian; and from an egg, Indian and Greek. The night sky was organized into constellations, and planets were observed and plotted by early astronomers. The earth was naturally taken as the center of the universe. Claudius Ptolemy, second century AD was the last of the great ancient astronomers. Conducting his observations in Alexandria, Egypt, he wrote a textbook of astronomy which was to be known as the Ptolemaic System. It represented the earth as stationary in the center of the universe with all other celestial objects moving about it in circular orbits.

This system was accepted for centuries until in 1593 the Polish astronomer and physician, Nicholas Copernicus, published his observations in his work, "Revolution of the Heaven and the Orbs." He observed looped rather than circular orbits of the planets and he described the sun as the center of the universe, with earth and planets moving about it. In 1609 the German astronomer and mathematician, Johann Kepler, refined and published Tyco Brahe's precise observation on the elliptical orbit of Mars and demonstrated that all other planets have elliptical orbits described by three basic principles. Kepler's laws are the application of the laws of physics to the motion of celestial bodies, the beginning of celestial mechanics. In 1609 Galileo constructed the first complete astronomical telescope. He discovered mountains on the moon and that the milky way consisted of many separate stars. He discovered Jupiter's four largest moons and their orbits. He discovered sun spots on the sun, the phases of Venus, and Saturn's indistinct rings. As a result of his observations and his public confirmation of the Copernican system he was subjected to arrest and lifetime confinement at the hands of the Inquisition.

Small variations in the planetary orbits motivated Isaac Newton in 1687 to develop his laws of motion and laws of universal gravitation. Albert Einstein's Relativity Theory, published in 1905, explains that gravity effects space and light as well as celestial bodies and redefines gravity as a warping of space by the mass of celestial bodies. During a total eclipse of the sun the apparent optical displacement of a star proved that massive celestial objects (the sun) does bend light by means of the warping of space. Einstein also proved that space and time are not constant but are determined by the location and motion of the observer. Einstein considered the universe to be static and eternal and therefore postulated a repulsive force, the cosmological constant to balance the field equations of universal gravitational collapse. Russian mathematician Alexander Friedman, in 1922, found other solutions to the Einstein gravitational field equations that showed the relativity theory to be compatible with an infinite expanding universe.

Belgium mathematician Georges Lemaitre, in 1927, postulated an explosive beginning for the expansion of the universe from a hot, dense "primeval atom" beginning which could be demonstrated by red shifts in astronomical observations. Edwin Hubbell and his astronomical assistant, Milton Humason observed nebulae to be distant galaxies like our own Milky Way galaxy, receding at red shifts speeds and proving the expansion of the universe. Physicist George Gamow published work in 1952 showing the forces of nuclear fusion and explosive big bang universe to be the source of inorganic complex physical elements, the building blocks of the physical universe. Radio astronomer Arno Penzias and Robert Wilson in 1965 detected microwave radiation in the sky which is a remnant of the beginning explosion of the big bang, the cosmic background radiation of the universe. In 1979 Alan Guth proposed that the early universe had an inflationary period in which it expanded rapidly, exceeding the speed of light, to account for its present immense size. In this theory Einstein's speed of light limited universe does not apply since the expansion of space itself is not the same as acceleration within created space.

Over billions of years the universe has evolved into varied and complex forms. Each second our universe expands by 186,000 miles, the speed of light. In 4 minutes an area the size of our Milky Way is created by expanding space. There are now hundreds of billions of galaxies, each with hundreds of billions of stars. Grand unified theories are proposed uniting the strong nuclear force, electro weak force, and gravity at very high energy levels presumed to exist at the beginning of the universe. Theories of cosmic super string, super symmetry and hyper space have been proposed in an effort to describe an unknown physics at the beginning of the universe. Physicist John Wheeler at the University of Texas proposes that this universe arose from a kind of cosmic foam with the specific qualities of space/time and the arbitrary physical laws which define our universe. He proposes many other universes can evolve from the unknown cosmic foam with different space/time parameters and different physical laws than our own universe. Of course there is no scientific proof for any of this theorizing but it serves to illustrate the unlimited possibilities. Another model of the universe is proposed by Dr. David Bohm, a physicist, and Dr. Karl Pibram, a neurophysiologist. In this model the universe is considered to be a hologram in which space, time, matter, energy and mind do not exist independently but are mental interpretations of relationships within a vast ocean of waves and frequencies. Interference patterns within this ocean, like those that produce holographic pictures, are responsible for the apparent appearance of all these properties of the universe.

So many theories indicate that there are undiscovered and unknown dimensions and states of existence in our vast and complex universe.

The totality of our so-called knowledge or beliefs,
from the most profound laws of atomic physics
or even mathematics and logic,
is a man-made fabric which impinges
on experience only along the edges.

W. V. L. Quine
Professor of Philosophy, Harvard University

Relativity and even more important,
quantum mechanics has strongly suggested
that the world cannot be analyzed into
separate and independently existing parts.
Moreover, each part somehow involves
all the others: contains and enfolds them.
This fact suggests that the sphere of
ordinary material life and the sphere of mystical
experience have a certain shared order and
that this will allow a fruitful
relationship between them.

David Bohm
Physics Professor, University of London

Chapter 8

Physical Phases and Transitions

Matter exists in three common ways we are all familiar with, solid, liquid and gas. There is a fourth unusual way matter can exist called plasma. A plasma is a gas produced at very high temperatures, thousands of degrees, composed of the nuclei of atoms stripped of their electrons. This mix of free negative electrons and positive nuclei is formed in stars. A less radical physical change is noted when matter changes between states of solid, liquid or gas. In each of these there is a change in structure but no change in chemical composition.

Changes in volume, pressure and temperature acting on the same substance can produce very different material. Carbon is the common atom in both graphite and diamond. Graphite is produced at low temperatures and pressures, diamond at high. Water a liquid, at high temperature becomes water vapor, a gas, and at colder temperatures changes to ice, a solid, with crystalline structure and symmetry. The phases of expression of the common molecule, H_2O depends on its internal energy. At high energy it's a gas, low energy a solid, medium energy a liquid. Glass is really a silica liquid because its molecules and atoms have not formed a stable crystalline pattern. A pane of glass left in place vertically for hundreds of years will show a flow downward in response to gravity. Very old European windows are thicker at the bottom than the top due to the liquid flow of glass over many years.

Not only can physical matter change into different states and still remain the same, but matter and energy can also change states between themselves, matter becoming energy and energy becoming matter. Matter becomes energy in thermonuclear reactions. In thermonuclear fission explosions a heavy element, uranium or plutonium splits into lighter elements, annihilating some of its mass and turning it into energy, $E=MC^2$.

Under controlled reactions of a nuclear power plant electricity (electromagnetic energy) is generated in this way. Within the sun thermonuclear fusion reactions continue to occur since its birth as a star five billion years ago. Nuclear fusion generates energetic photon energy called gamma radiation. As gamma rays work their way through the rest of the sun's mass they are absorbed and readmitted as two photons of lower energy. After many such absorption's and re-admissions the life giving photons of sunlight which we see, feel and absorb on earth are produced.

In the photosphere of the sun, hydrogen atoms capture free electrons which produce photons of light. These electrons captured at different energy levels produce the electromagnetic spectrum, a portion of which is visible light. Each day the earth, including every living thing on it, absorbs a total of several pounds of sunlight photons. In this way the sun accomplishes the transition of a part of itself into life. Through nucleosynthesis at the core of every star including the sun, elements of matter, up to iron, are produced. As heavy stars (multiples of the suns mass) super nova (explode) at the end of their life cycle, these lighter elements of nature are fused to produce all the heavier elements of nature. Out of all these elements life forms evolve. Organic bodies of life phase into existence from inanimate inorganic sources of nature. Basic inorganic matter, the subatomic particles of neutrons, electrons, and protons are created when energy becomes matter.

Particle physicists have to date discovered hundreds of subatomic particles, and some, protons and neutrons are explained by the theory of quantum chromodynamics and quark combinations. Six quarks combine in doublets or in triplets to form primary subatomic nuclear particles. A quark is a subatomic particle which has dimension and responds to the strong nuclear force. The strong nuclear force in turn is carried by the mediator particle, the gluon. Subatomic elementary particles which do not respond to the strong nuclear force and have no numerical dimension such as the electron and neutrinos, are called leptons. The combination of leptons and quarks are responsible for all the created matter as explained by the current standard model of matter. However, the most essential property of matter, it's mass, has yet to be adequately explained.

A mass bestowing particle of immense electron voltage has been suggested to exist. This has been named the Higgs boson, but no laboratory has been able to detect it.

A competing theory, the S-matrix or bootstrap theory, holds that matter cannot be reduced to ultimate basic subatomic particles. Matter and nature altogether is a dynamic interactive relationship of events within the matrix of physical existence. No part is fundamental and all take their characteristics and properties from their relationship with the other parts. The theory is a self consistent, self contained description of all possible particle interactions beginning from the origin of the universe. The standard model describes the origin of matter at the beginning of the universe differently. At the big bang origin highly energetic radiation photons are produced at high temperatures and pressures not reproducible on earth. As the explosion cools slightly these photons unite to produce particles and anti particle pairs of quarks, leptons, electrons, protons, neutrons, neutrinos. Some pairs annihilate themselves back into radiation energy.

There is a vast excess of particles over anti particles, or matter over anti matter for unknown reasons, perhaps due to pair splitting by black holes in which most anti particles disappear and the subatomic particles that remain coalesce and eventually form the matter of the universe as it exists today. Radiation energy from the origin of the universe has created matter. Visible matter is only a small part of the matter created. Scientists believe that most of the matter in the universe is dark unseen matter responsible for galaxy formation and gravitational discrepancies (the gravitational constant) and the missing mass of the universe.

In addition some scientists and mathematicians believe that there are more dimensions to reality than the accepted ones of three of space and one of time. Hidden dimensions higher than four are invoked to help explain the unification of the fundamental forces of nature; strong nuclear force, electro weak force, gravity and to explain the non-locality problem of quantum theory.

The non-locality qualities of the quantum material world support the existence of extra dimensions beyond the four dimensions of the everyday world. Einstein called it spooky action at a distance which indicated hidden variables working at the level of quantum matter. This phenomenon is demonstrated when paired particles of matter (protons, electrons or photons) are separated by vast distances, but can still communicate information instantaneously without passing through the intervening space. Experiments by Allen Aspect, Leonard Mandel at the University of Rochester, and Raymond Chiao at the University of California all demonstrate this faster than light phenomenon to be real at the quantum level of existence. David Bohm, Einstein's protegé, explained this phenomenon in his theory of the implicate order of things.

Dr. Bohm theorizes that in the implicate order all things in the universe including quantum particles, and macroscopic particles are interconnected and communicate with each other. Dr. Bohm suggests that any particles that once were in contact with each other would continue to be able to communicate with each other even when separated by vast distances. Some scientists suggest that large distances in our ordinary four dimensional space/time world could be reduced to very short distances in the reality of a universe of higher dimensions than four. Higher dimensions are also considered to be necessary when theorizing about the unification of the separate forces of nature into one unified force.

When the strong nuclear force, electro weak force, and gravity are united in a grand unified theory, spatial dimensions higher than four are required to mathematically demonstrate the unification. Finally, extra unseen dimensions are suggested to have application in the inflationary model of the expansion of the universe. At an early stage of development the universe expanded extremely rapidly, creating the vast space of the universe, utilizing faster than light speed. Superluminal or tachyonic speed is not possible in Einstein's space/time continuum world, but is possible in a universe of higher dimensions than the four of space and time.

The science of topology is a branch of mathematics that addresses the structure of curved space. Topological properties remain constant while experiencing continuous distortions of space. A part of spatial topology called cohomology concerns the patching together of varying spatial geometrics. An example is artist M.C. Escher's drawings of spatially incongruous subjects in multiple planes. In cohomology space encoded structures can then become manifest differently within a varied expansive geometry without losing their essential characteristics.

A variant of complex topological space called twister space was developed by mathematician Roger Penrose which was capable of uniting the four fundamental forces of nature and matter. Objects in twister space are not points but one dimensional objects extended in space represented by the complex number of generalized light rays. This concept became even more impressive when it was united with another recent development of physics called string theory. In string theory matter does not obey the cause and effect laws of classical Newtonian physics but only at the very small subquantum distances of 10^{-33} centimeters or Planks distance. At this distance the quarks which unite in triplets to form protons and neutrons and therefore atomic nuclei, are not point particles but are considered the lowest vibration of tiny strings. Super strings can be open, closed, or looped, and thereby can also accommodate the four fundamental forces of nature as primary string vibrations. Ten or more basic dimensions of original space spontaneously compactify down to 4 on the macroscopic level.

A combination of twister and cohomological space with complex string effects can explain unseen qualities of nature within a very complex and unknown cosmic topology. Such a cosmic topology could conceal spiritual existence.

When we come to light we are
coming to the fundamental activity
in which existence has it's ground.
Light is the potential of everything.

David Bohm

All of consciousness arises in
dependence in this mind of clear light.

Dali Lama

Light is the shadow of God.

Plato

Chapter 9

Light

Albert Einstein's Relativity theory unifies space and time into the single entity of space/time. He reasoned that matter and energy could also be related according to relativity. The mass of an object increases as it accelerates and he concluded that the increase in mass comes from the energy of speed. The conservation of mass and the conservation of energy in a closed system was uniformly accepted by physicists of the time and now he stated that the sum total of the mass and the sum total of the energy always remains the same as well. The result it his famous equation $E=MC^2$.

Since the speed of light C is 186,000 miles per second, C squared is a huge number and the amount of energy contained in a small amount of matter is therefore, enormous. Light is an integral part of both mass and energy. Einstein's formula applied Max Plank's quantum theory at the source of thermal radiation (black body radiation) to the radiation itself, stating that light and other electromagnetic radiation travels in discrete tiny bundles which he named light quanta or photons. This concept aided his investigation into the photo electric effect and supported the concept of light as a particle as proposed by Newton 250 years ago. Light also demonstrated the phenomenon of reflection/refraction, defraction, interference and polarization, all of which are best explained by the wave theory of light proposed by Christian Huygens in 1690.

Light is now considered to be both wave and particle. The particle properties predominate when photons are emitted or absorbed by substances, and the wave properties predominate when light is transmitted or propagated. In 1924, Louis de Broglie extended this concept to matter, proposing that moving particles have wave properties similar to light. Matter and energy, wave and particles are all related in some way to qualities of light, the quintessential wave particle duality. Light is one of the most ubiquitous components of the universe. Visible light is a small portion of a wide energy spectrum (the electromagnetic spectrum) and is visible to us only because of the size and design of the human eye. Light has some very peculiar qualities. A light photon at rest has no mass, no space, and no energy. It does not exist except that when it is in motion it acquires a kinetic moving mass and a kinetic moving energy. A light photon has no electrical charge. Objects that travel at relativistic speeds, (approaching the speed of light, 186,000 miles per second) gain enormously in mass and shrink dramatically in dimension.

Time itself slows and ultimately stops when the speed of light is reached. Light is a fundamental determinate of the universe. In addition, light is its own anti matter particle. Photons existed as electromagnetic radiation at the universe's big bang, and some theoretical physicists feel that the universe originated from a primordial vacuum (void) by means of a quantum fluctuation in a field of virtual photons producing the matter and energy of the universe at the point of singularity origin. Photons outnumber protons of matter, two billion to one, in our present universe. Some scientists theorize that matter is actually frozen or trapped photons.

Recently a physics professor at Cologne University, Germany, has succeeded in demonstrating the faster than light capability of quantum waves. He encoded music onto a type of laser beam which then tunneled through a barrier in his laboratory. He calculated that the photon waves of light traveled five times faster than the accepted absolute light speed of 186,000 miles per second.

Light interacts with bodies in many ways, the suntan and warmth on the beach, the colors and shapes our eye perceives, hormonal circadian rhythms of the brain are a few of the effects of light on the human body. The proteins, enzymes and DNA of our own bodies are active absorbers of visible and invisible light. All twenty amino acids from which proteins are formed are optically active and can rotate the plane of polarized light, depending on the asymmetry of their chiral centers. Living cells and organisms release weak photon emission, different from bioluminescence when they die. As reported by scientists Fritz Albert Popp, and Frohlich and Kremer, large living organisms emit a death flash of light upon dying.

Researchers at Wellman Laboratory of Harvard University, Drs. Stephen Jacques, David Weaver, and Steven Reppert demonstrated that visible light in the range of 400 (blue) to 650 (pale red), and invisible light below 400 nanometers penetrate through the intact abdomen of pregnant guinea pigs and is recorded by fiber optic detectors inside the pregnant uterus containing a developing fetus. The rate of light transmission and absorption is very low, but a real value. Light visible and invisible can reach developing fetuses. By extrapolation it would appear to apply to humans as well. Light and life are intricately associated.

Light has an integral contribution at every level of physical existence. For example, at the molecular level of matter, light amplified and stimulated (LASER) radiation creates a plasma of energy which breaks apart the molecules of the target. This is the method used in laser surgery to remove pathological tissue.

At the atomic level, light quantum absorption and emission is required for the electron to jump or fall back to another orbital plane about the nucleus. The quantum jump is responsible for the quantum ladder of the atomic electron and is how laser light is produced. Light quantum absorption is responsible for the photoelectric effect in which sufficiently strong light of 3.5 electron volts or higher (deep blue or violet or ultraviolet) when shown upon certain metals, strips free electrons from the outer orbits of the atoms producing a flow of electrons or an electrical current. Solar energy devices produce electricity in a similar manner.

Photons of light energy are responsible for certain radioactive activity as demonstrated by the recent union of the weak nuclear force and the electromagnetic force into the second united field force of nature, the electro weak force. It is calculated that the electro weak photon unification occurs at energies of 100 billion electron volts. It is theorized that at energies of 10^{15} billion electron volts the strong and electro weak photons are united into a single force which in turn unifies with the final universal force of gravity at 10^{19} billion electron volts. These enormous energies and this final unification is theorized to occur when the universe was at 10^{-43} seconds old. This time frame has been named Plank time in honor of the German physicist Max Plank, who discovered the basic quantum and black body radiation theories. The history of the universe after this time evolves following the rules established by Einstein, and according to his theory of relativity. Prior to Plank's time the physics of the very early universe is unknown. An unknown universe could encompass anything, including spiritual existence.

Part IV

Spiritual Paradigm

Losing Personality

Birth Spirit - Existential Spirit

An Existential Paradigm

A Better Humanity

Whatever we
might think of this world,
it is astonishing.

Wislowa Szymborska
Nobel Prize in Literature 1996

Chapter 10

Losing Personality

As we have seen, personality is the external demonstration of the self identity evolved from experience, choices, family environment, and genes. My relatives have told me that on occasion, in my youth, they have seen a very intense brilliant light filling my bedroom when I was sleeping. When I awaken in the morning following such a night I find that my everyday personality is different. Gone are the little idiosyncrasies and quirks. Limited points of view are replaced with global ones. A panoramic view of life is appreciated, and thinking is simple, uncluttered, unpretentious and clear. The emotion of agape replaces all others. There is a feeling of purpose and design for humanity and the world. I know that everything that exists and everyone who exists is sacred.

On two such occasions I noticed in the morning the presence of a few unusual spots on the floor about the foot and side of the bed. These were uniform, tan, gelatinous, amorphous, odorless masses, sometimes an inch or so in diameter and half as thick. They are usually in large droplet form, but one in particular, the largest, was swirled-looking, like the top of soft ice cream from a nozzle dispenser. The personality is specific for each person, defining that person and, I believe intimately and physically associated with the physical body. To me, these drops are my shedded, faulted personality. There is a phenomenon called cellular memory which I believe is related.

Cellular memory is the label that has been applied to the reports of many recipients of organ transplants. Solid organs of the body; heart, lung, liver, kidney, are harvested from donors, usually who have a tragic end. Patients with severe diseases affecting these organs receive the donor's organs and sometimes more than one organ at the same time. Heart and lungs are transplanted as a unit, liver, stomach and intestines transplanted as a unit similarly. There is a great amount of tissue weighing several pounds transplanted, all of which has been kept alive by perfusion and cooling since the time it was harvested from the donor. When some of the organ recipients awakened from anesthesia post-operatively and in the recovery period, they report changes in their own personality. Different cravings for food and drink, different habits and preferences which were later found to match the food and drink preferences or habits of the deceased donors. In other words, some of the personality traits of the donor had appeared in the recipient's now changed post-operative personality. Science explains the phenomenon as either a reaction to post-operative potent anti rejection drugs like steroids or to psychological processes in the recipients seeking stress resolution or wishes of appreciation and identification with the donor.

My personal experience leads me to believe that due to the very large amount of tissue and DNA being transplanted, some physically dependent basic personality traits are also transplanted. If the recipient has inherent qualities of sensitivity they will perceive these effects, others less sensitive will not.

There is another example of losing personality occuring in clinical medicine. The end of life for patients with incurable terminal diseases can sometimes contain experiences of loss of personality.

Dr. Elizabeth Kubler Ross, in her book "On Death and Dying" - Macmillan Press, describes five stages of psychological processes that terminal patients experience in an effort to reach mental equilibrium once they realize that their life is coming to an end. The first stage is denial. "It can't be true, it can't happen to me". The second is anger, "Why should it be me? I do not deserve to die." Third is bargaining, "Perhaps I can exhort the doctor to give me the medical miracle he is hiding from me", or "Perhaps God will save me if in turn I change certain things about myself." Fourthly, depression, "None of these things are going to happen. I am doomed." Fifth, acceptance, "I am worn out and can't resist the inevitable."

Sometimes during these stages doctors see a different response from the patient. The patient feels that this process of dying is not happening to him, not to the true actual "me". "It is happening to someone else, distant from me." A split in consciousness can occur at this moment and the patient recognizes, perhaps for the first time in his life, that the body and personality that he has all along felt to be his complete self, is not in fact his complete self. There is a break in identity following which he identifies most closely with this other self, this non-physical, spiritual self.

For the doctor this event appears to be a medical emergency. The patient has developed an identity crisis. He has lost his personality and this, the doctor has been taught, is psychologically pathological. The patient has de-personalized, a hallmark of a severe psychiatric disease or psychosis. A well identified, sound personality is essential for a lifetime of healthy living and we have examined some of these personality formation theories earlier. But now at the end of earthly life the parameters of survival are shifting, and a new paradigm of existence is beginning to emerge.

This process of de-personalization can disturb and distress the unprepared doctor. He decides to ask for a psychiatric evaluation. The psychiatrist tries to help the patient re-identify with his earthly persona. This I believe is a tragic mistake for the well-being of the patient. The patient's body will die in any case and since he has now finally recognized the existence of a continuing spirit, his spiritual core being, he should be allowed to complete the death transition process undisturbed.

His conscious feelings and memories will continue to exist spiritually when death is finished and he should be given time to become comfortable with this change in phase existence. As the two deaths I have attended demonstrate, this spiritual transition occurs with a substantive spiritual material body of light continuing to survive.

The world does not require so much
to be informed as to be reminded.

Hannah More

Beauty is merely the spiritual
making itself known sensually.

Georg Hagel

Chapter 11

Birth Spirit — Existential Spirit

About ten million babies are born into the world each month. Examination of newborns shortly after birth shows them to possess a little understood phenomenon. A newborn typically is extremely short-sighted but outgrows this as the eye and body progress. The focusing resolution of vision at this time is only a few inches from the infant's face. When an examiner places his face within this range of vision, the infant will mimic the tongue position changes that it sees the examiner perform. In a matter of hours this capability disappears. What is happening here?

I have retained conscious knowledge and memory of my own birth. I had a great desire and longing for re-birth. In an intermediate pre-birth period, an unknown matching process occurred with occasional openings appearing in a cloudy veil showing couples in love. One of these couples was my parents and I saw them walking hand-in-hand with joyful loving eyes, and surrounded in love. Spiritual friends had questioned me about why I wanted to be born again as they were very apprehensive, feeling that the earth is a very challenging and dangerous place. Just before birth, my birth spirit saw a luminous globe of interconnected potential events representing all the potential paths of the coming life. The choices made during life would determine the actual kinetic reality of the summed life about to begin.

There was a very short time in which my birth spirit reflected upon itself, asking who am I about to make this transition? It saw itself as intelligent and purposeful to the point of wisdom. It saw a long prior history of existence more ancient than ancient, without a discernible starting point. It felt that the new birth step it was taking was to be a great exhilarating spiritual adventure, joyfully entering it with a deep sense of purpose and mission. As the moment of birth approached, my birth spirit felt itself being pulled rapidly into the infant being born. It tried unsuccessfully to slow the process down, feeling loss of control. The next moment, it was inside the newborn and realized that it was alive again. It quickly accepted the newborn as its new home and settled into it cozily with an over-riding feeling of secure love.

Following this, during the first days of life, the infant sleeps constantly and it is during this time that birth spirit normally loses its memory, becoming overwhelmed by the physicality and the senses of the newborn. It becomes identified totally with the baby. In the first few hours of life, before a total identification, that newborn tongue mimicking phenomenon hints at the intelligent spirit that has entered at birth and which will be shortly overwhelmed by the physical state. The vast majority of people do not remember any of this, only a few will remember their original birth spirit. I believe everyone who was born had this process occur at birth. The loss of it's memory may be the cause of the spiritual search for meaning and identity that concerns many people later on in life.

I have also retained conscious knowledge and memory of spiritual states of existence before any of this occurred. When my birth spirit decided to be reborn, it was approached by spiritual beings whom I call "friends". They were apprehensive about my decision, feeling that life on earth was dangerous, full of confusion and misdirection. These spiritual beings exist in a state of primeness. They are all highly developed spiritual beings, not in human form but as bright luminous spiritual bodies. These primed spiritual beings are intelligent, compassionate, wise and full of the emotion of universal agape. They prefer to assist by spiritual means rather than by physical presence. Their state of existence is one of brilliant ecstasy and beauty. They are all of the same kind of highly developed spiritual mind. There is no flawed thinking, reasoning, or emotion in them. This allows them to fully appreciate each other's spirit and mind which they freely share with each other in a kind of spiritual communion.

There is another state of existence which I consider to be the ultimate state, the supreme source of all being and becoming. It may appear to be a state of non-existence, but it is much greater than that. In it there is no self-identified spirit because a spiritual being capable of entering into it is completely dissolved in it. There remains no boundary, no border delineating the entering spirit. The ultimate state is the ground origin of being, the ground origin of existence itself, existential spirit. It is oceanic, awesome in power, mind and agape, dynamically compassionate and beautiful beyond description. A spiritual being drawn into it is in a constant state of ecstasy and beauty, devoid of thought.

At some unknown point a precipitation of individual spirit spontaneously occurs. The spiritual being is reformed and reborn, now full of creative energy. It has an inborn need to participate in the eternal flow of beauty called existence. Non use of this creative energy, born from the source sickens and weakens the spirit. The reborn spirit knows that creative growth and the diversity of expression of being, the flowering of being is paramount to the source. The spiritual being therefore participates in the process according to the options available to it. The available options depend upon the sum spiritual state of the individual spiritual being.

There is a third spiritual state which is very broad and contains a wide range of spiritual beings. All are mentally confused in one way or another. Some are obsessed by thoughts and desires of power, wealth, money, sex, and controlling others for personal gain. These desires cannot be satisfied spiritually. These spirits all seek rebirth on earth quickly in an effort to physically express and satisfy these desires.

There is another drive for human birth and that is the desire for the security of physicality. The physical reference point of the human body is necessary for some spiritual beings who doubt their own non physical spiritual existence. Confused spiritual minds need to return to earth and work out their confusion.

*In the good,
the beautiful, the true,
we see reality revealing
it's personal character.*

Rudolph Eucken
Nobel Prize in Literature 1908

Chapter 12

An Existential Paradigm

By now, an existential paradigm may be delineated from the preceding. I have attempted to show the essential, basic and significant part light contributes in nature, from the origin of the universe to the subatomic and macroscopic levels of physical reality. The clinical patient events I have described reveal the true nature of the human spirit to also have some characteristics of light albeit a different kind of light, a spiritual light. The dualistic theory of separate mind and spirit from the body is reinforced. Materialists' theory of mind, identity and consciousness being solely derived from brain tissue is not supported.

Personality has been shown to depend greatly on genetics, on the neurophysical and neurochemical, and psychosocial activity of the brain. Personality is not identical with the birth human spirit but utilized as a temporal operational mode by existential spirit. Descriptions of the mysteries of quantum theory, string theory, twister topological space, and cohomology space, suggest the possibility of faster than light communications and hidden dimensions of reality beyond four. Existential spirit could pass into and out of our spatial world through the cohomologous interface portal. This is supported by the clinical events I have experienced.

We are all born with an original birth spirit. The physicalness of a body and the creation of a personality quickly overwhelm our knowledge and memory of birth spirit. Much less do we remember the existential spirit from which all birth spiritual beings originate.

We are the creators, experiencers and recorders of our individual life experiences and altogether are creating and recording the entire experiential phenomenon of humanity. The activity of confused and sick willful personalities cause much suffering for humanity. Personality is physically and mentally dependent on the human condition. Spiritual beings progress during life, survive death, and may access higher spiritual states of being when capable. The surviving spiritual being records and relives all the events of its earthly life, feeling the pain and anguish it inflicts, as well as the joy and agape nature of almost everything else. The surviving spiritual being harvests the joy and agape and contributes to the eternal flowing beauty of existential being.

The universe is complex and continues to have many unknowns, but is it probably finite and therefore one day, will end, just as the earth and humanity will. What continues eternally is the flowing beauty and agape of existential being, of which a human life is a creative part.

Scientists attempt to explain mystical experiences as abnormal electrical activity of the temporal or frontal cortex of the brain, or as hallucinations. They also suggest that in terminal physical states, the reduction of blood flow to various parts of the brain can produce visual hallucinations or visions without basis in reality. Being able to perform a surgical procedure, such as the delivery of a baby, tying and cutting the umbilical cord, and assisting in suturing of the surgical episiotomy cannot be performed while under the effects of visual hallucinations or temporal lobe brain dysfunction. There is no doubt in my mind that all the personal experiences I have related here are real events.

The material contained here is bound to be controversial. Some people will be able to understand and accept it, and learn from it. Others will not be able to. Some will oppose what I have related. Opponents, rivals and adversaries are common in life. If the real significance of the adversarial process is recognized, we can appreciate the relationship for its basic sacredness. An adversary is sacred because the adversarial position offers the opportunity for spiritual growth. Typically an escalation of rationalized negative thinking and action occurs between opponents. You said this or did that which offended me, therefore I am justified in saying this or doing that to you.

Sometimes the battle occurs indirectly by trying to weaken or destroy the adversary's base of operation, or support. The winner of such a controversy may feel vindicated, but also generates for himself heavy negative emotional thinking and memory. These negatively impact the person's spirit and later will be re-experienced spiritually, but this time with positions reversed. However if the process is recognized when it happens, it can be cut off at the root.

Mind and emotion can be tamed in this way; by becoming aware of our own thought processes we can see how our mind works and what the likely outcome will be. With this insight we can exert an active will to change the process into one of understanding and empathy. The adversarial situation is therefore instrumental in acquiring this new quality of being able to turn negative thinking and emotion into positive ones. Subsequently this approach can be utilized in many other life situations, to help refine not only the mind and emotions, but ultimately the spirit.

For all sad words of tongue or pen,
the saddest are these:
"It might have been."

John Greenleaf Whittier

Chapter 13

A Better Humanity

I believe humanity can be improved from it's current condition. Advances in medical science can enhance both the beginning and the ending of life.

It is my opinion that the struggle and suffering that so often accompanies a person's death in the final weeks and days of a terminal illness can be avoided. The two deaths that I have observed were without suffering and very peaceful. They both occurred under the conditions and circumstances of a clinical coma. I propose that when a terminal illness is causing uncontrollable pain or discomfort for a patient, a medical coma can be induced and maintained until the final passing peacefully occurs. A legal document can be created that a seriously ill patient with full mental faculties can sign, authorizing such treatment if it becomes necessary. Hospitals commonly have legal forms that a critical patient can sign appointing a health care surrogate to make final health care decisions, such as "do not resuscitate" orders if the patient becomes mentally and physically incapacitated during a hospitalization. An agreement to include a final coma order could also be added to these documents. Only after several doctors evaluate the patient, and agree that the patient is terminal and suffering despite pain management, would such an order be executed. Terminal pain or suffering serves no good purpose and society should allow the next state of spiritual existence to begin peacefully.

As the ending of life can be improved, the beginning of life can also be improved by medical science. Advanced medical research has demonstrated the ability to isolate embryonic stem cells from the blastocyst stage of early human embryo development. At this laboratory stage, the approximately 100 cell embryo has formed an inner cell mass and an outer cell mass. The outer cell mass will develop into the placenta and amniotic sac of the embryo only if it is implanted into the lining of a prepared and receptive woman's uterus. The inner cell mass will develop into the body of the fetus. Human embryo research is currently very controversial but holds the answer to vast health improvements for all people. When the outer cell mass is dissolved in the laboratory, the inner call mass, which is no longer able to form a survivable embryo, can be chemically induced to grow and to differentiate into various cell tissue colonies. Heart, muscle, nerve, cartilage, pancreas and liver cells are among those already produced which can then be injected into a patient who has a disease of one of these organs. If the patient's own nuclear chromosome material is placed by intracystoplasmic injection into an egg cell which has had it's native nuclear material removed, the resulting embryonic stem cells will develop cells and tissues which are completely compatible with the patient. Transplant and implant rejection will be impossible and the patient will be cured.

Similar manipulations of the human egg and sperm cells can result in complete human clones, again a very controversial subject. A modified cloning technique may be able in the near future to dramatically improve the human condition. The human Genome project is today deciphering the nucleotide base sequencing for each of the 80,000 to 100,000 genes located in the human chromosome. DNA is the active molecule in the chromosome. The genes are distributed throughout the DNA molecule in segments, in code for the cellular synthesis of proteins and enzymes. DNA is a long but extremely thin, biological molecule. Each cell in the body has six feet of it coiled up within the cell nucleus. Laid end-to-end, all the DNA in the 250 billion cells of a single person's body would stretch for hundreds of thousands of miles. Errors in nucleotide base sequencing during DNA division and duplication are called mutations and cause inherited disease through the abnormal production of proteins and enzymes. Errors in the deciphering of the DNA code by the cell's messenger RNA also result in disease. Hundreds of human diseases and afflictions have been traced to these errors.

Gene therapy is already indicating it's enormous potential for humanity. Recently, research scientists have been able to insert a gene for the protein catalytic component of telomerase into the cell nucleus. The telomere is a nuclear structure essential in accomplishing mitosis or the replication of cells. Aging cells show progressively less telemere structure as they divide. Ultimately, without a telomere they can no longer divide and die. By adding catalytic telomerase, the telomere is replenished and cell division returns to youthful levels. The young cells produced by this method in the laboratory are completely normal. This is a major step towards reversing the aging process.

Another gene project in Iceland will determine the sequencing differences between healthy and diseased genes. The entire population of Iceland is participating and was selected because this country has the most homogenous hereditary line in the human population. When these two projects are completed, we will have the basic knowledge necessary to genetically engineer out most, or perhaps all, of the diseases and personality flaws afflicting humanity. Physical, emotional, and mental illness can finally be eliminated, resulting in a disease-free, healthy body, mind, and personality. Then, the golden age of humanity will dawn over the entire planet.

There is a love like a small lamp,
which goes out when the oil is consumed;
or like a stream, which dries up when it
doesn't rain. But there is a love that is
like a mighty spring gushing
up out of the earth;
it keeps flowing forever,
and is inexhaustible.

Isaac of Nineveh

We lie in the lap of immense intelligence,
which makes us receivers of its
truth and organs of its activity.

Ralph Waldo Emerson

Appendix

Love, Truth and Beauty

At the height of ancient Greek culture, more than 2000 years ago, love was described in three ways. The first was ***eros,*** or the physical love of sensual attraction. The second was ***philios*** or ***filios***, the love of friendship or platonic love. The third was ***agape***, a transcendent universal form of love for all creation. Each type was a refined order of love derived in part from the preceding love. The attainment of agapic love was then and still is today, the epitome of loving emotion and is closely allied with empathy and compassion. It is the spiritual emotion which contains in itself, all truth and beauty. Walt Whitman wrote: ***"truth is whatever satisfies the soul."***

By inference, agapic truth is whatever satisfies universal spirit. Truth also has the aspect of beauty inherent in it. The element of beauty is contained within existential spirit. Many things in this universe of existence are beautiful. The form and symmetry of matter in living things demonstrate it. Patterns of beauty are represented generously in nature. The orbit of celestial bodies, the spirals of the galaxies, including our own Milky Way galaxy, the spirals of shellfish and the spirals of the DNA molecule. The cycles of water, oxygen and carbon dioxide on earth and the circadian rhythms and hormone cycles within our bodies. All are examples of the beauty of existence. Paul Dirac, mathematician and Noble Laureate, stated that only beautiful mathematical formulas adequately described how nature worked. If a less beautiful formula was applied it was always subsequently found to be inferior to the more beautiful formula.

Chaos also, is present in the universe. Galaxies collide and cause redistribution of stars and matter. Our own galaxy is at this time colliding with the outer fringes of another smaller galaxy. Large stars explode into super novae and redistribute the elements created in its nuclear fusion furnace at its center. Planets are formed in the great crucible of hot, amorphous discs of matter surrounding stars. Hurricanes, tornadoes, and earthquakes occur on the earth as it attempts to rebalance the huge opposing forces working within it. Chaos theory states that seen from another dimension of observation, chaos is a process in the creation of higher order.

We are unable to appreciate this process because of our intimacy and proximity to it. Beauty exists all around us if we can become aware of its presence. By becoming aware of its presence the universe knows itself through us. Humankind can create beauty through all the kinds of expression of our intelligent mind. Humans are agents of beauty and as such participate in the nature of existential spirit.

All these: agape, truth and beauty, empathy and compassion, are the core qualities of the universal spiritual source, the source of all being and the cause of all becoming. Becoming is the truth that satisfies and embodies universal existential spirit.

BIRTH SPIRIT ENTERING

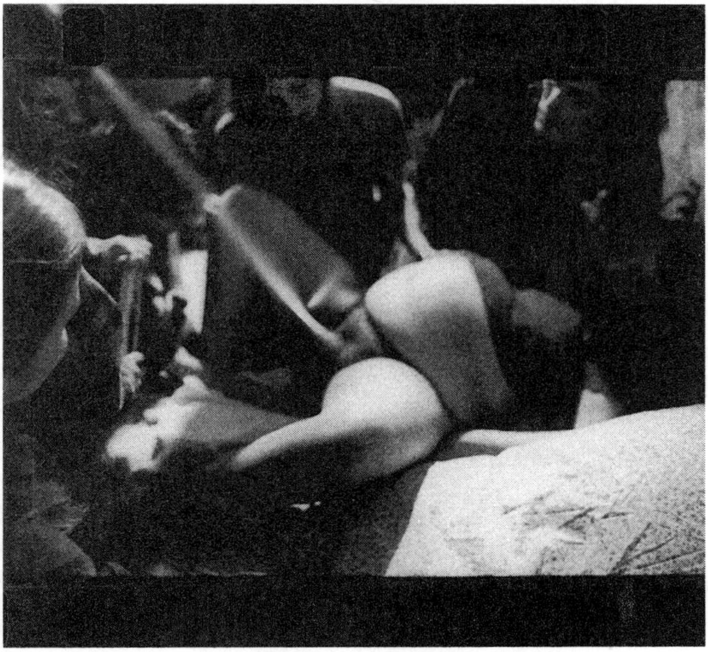

Photo Credit: Daniel A. Brown

Invocation of Birth Spirit

In preparation, find a quiet place away from everyday concerns. A sanctuary area in your home is ideal, but any quiet place will suffice.

Next, use the relaxation technique of your choice. If you have none, the following is suggested. Sit on a chair leaning slightly forward, so that your back does not rest against the chair-back. Do not lean so forward as to feel unbalanced on the chair.

Start by consciously relaxing the muscle tension in your toes, then feet, then slowly up your lower legs, than upper legs, stomach, back, chest, arms, hands, neck and head. Be conscious of your entire body glowing in comfort and peace. Next, clear your mind of all thoughts of worldly concerns by picturing in your mind, a clear glowing light. Then, proceed as follows on the next page.